INTRODUCTION TO CLINICAL RESEARCH FUNDAMENTALS

A Comprehensive Guide for Beginners

Dr Essam Abdelhakim

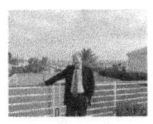

Copyright © 2024 Dr Essam Abdelhakim

All rights reserved

The characters and events portrayed in this book are fictitious. Any similarity to real persons, living or dead, is coincidental and not intended by the author.

No part of this book may be reproduced, or stored in a retrieval system, or transmitted in any form or by any means, electronic, mechanical, photocopying, recording, or otherwise, without express written permission of the publisher.

Cover design by: Art Painter
Library of Congress Control Number: 2018675309
Printed in the United States of America

CONTENTS

Title Page
Copyright
Chapter 1: Introduction to Clinical Research — 1
Chapter 2: Research Ethics and Regulatory Frameworks — 5
Chapter 3: Study Design Basics — 10
Chapter 4: Data Collection and Management — 15
Chapter 5: Statistical Foundations for Beginners — 21
Chapter 6: Writing and Publishing Your Research — 27
Chapter 7: Challenges and Pitfalls in Clinical Research — 32
Chapter 8: Future Trends in Clinical Research — 37
Appendices — 42
About The Author — 47

CHAPTER 1: INTRODUCTION TO CLINICAL RESEARCH

What is Clinical Research?
Definitions and Key Concepts:
Clinical research is a branch of healthcare science that focuses on understanding diseases, developing treatments, and improving health outcomes by studying human participants.

It encompasses studies that test new treatments, observe health conditions, or evaluate healthcare interventions.

Key components of clinical research include:

1. **Human Participants:** The central focus is on individuals, whether healthy or affected by a condition.
2. **Scientific Methodology:** Research is conducted systematically to ensure reliable results.
3. **Outcomes:** The goal is to improve understanding, prevention, diagnosis, or treatment of diseases.

For instance, a clinical trial may explore the safety and efficacy of a new cancer drug, while an observational study might investigate the long-term effects of diabetes on cardiovascular health.

Differences Between Clinical And Basic Research:

While both types of research are crucial for advancing healthcare, they differ significantly in focus and methods:

Aspect	Clinical Research	Basic Research
Focus	Studies human	Explores fundamental

	participants and interventions	biological processes
Objective	Improves patient care and treatments	Expands theoretical knowledge
Setting	Conducted in hospitals, clinics, or field	Performed in laboratories
Examples	Drug trials, epidemiological studies	Cell biology, genetics, molecular studies

Basic research often informs clinical research, providing foundational insights that later translate into real-world applications.

Importance Of Clinical Research In Healthcare

Advancing Medical Knowledge:
Clinical research bridges the gap between theoretical understanding and practical application.
By studying diseases in humans, researchers:
- Identify disease mechanisms.
- Develop diagnostic tools.
- Validate treatment efficacy.

Improving Patient Care And Outcomes:

Through rigorous testing, clinical research ensures that medical interventions are safe and effective.
- **Quality of Life:** Research evaluates therapies to enhance patient well-being.
- **Personalized Medicine:** Trials focus on tailoring treatments to individual genetic or environmental factors.

Types Of Clinical Research

Observational Studies vs. Interventional Trials:
Clinical research can broadly be categorized based on the level of researcher involvement:

Type	Definition	Examples
Observational Study	Researchers observe outcomes without intervening.	Cohort studies, case-control studies
Interventional Trial	Researchers actively introduce an intervention and measure its effect.	Drug trials, surgical interventions

Observational Studies:

- Explore associations between risk factors and outcomes.
- Generate hypotheses for further testing.
- Example: A cohort study investigating smoking as a risk factor for lung cancer.

Interventional Trials:

- Test specific treatments or interventions.
- Include a control group for comparison.
- Example: A randomized controlled trial (RCT) assessing a new vaccine.

Examples Of Study Designs:

1. **Randomized Controlled Trials (RCTs):**
    - Gold standard for testing interventions.
    - Participants are randomly assigned to treatment or control groups to reduce bias.
    - Example: Testing a new diabetes drug against a placebo.
2. **Cohort Studies:**
    - Follow a group with a shared characteristic over time to observe outcomes.
    - Example: Monitoring heart disease development in patients with high cholesterol.
3. **Case-Control Studies:**
    - Compare individuals with a condition (cases) to those without (controls).
    - Example: Identifying risk factors for breast cancer by comparing affected and unaffected women.
4. **Cross-Sectional Studies:**
    - Analyze data at a single point in time.
    - Example: Surveying a population to determine the prevalence of hypertension.

CHAPTER 2: RESEARCH ETHICS AND REGULATORY FRAMEWORKS

Ethics is a cornerstone of clinical research, ensuring the safety, dignity, and rights of participants.

The History Of Research Ethics

The development of research ethics was shaped by historical events that highlighted the need for guidelines to protect participants from harm.

1. The Nuremberg Code (1947):
- Origin: Developed after the Nuremberg Trials, where Nazi doctors were prosecuted for conducting inhumane experiments during World War II.
- Key Points:
  - **Voluntary Consent:** Participation must be informed and voluntary.
  - **Beneficence:** Experiments should aim to yield benefits for society and avoid unnecessary suffering.
  - **Right to Withdraw:** Participants can withdraw at any time.

2. Declaration of Helsinki (1964, with updates):
- Issued by the World Medical Association to provide a framework for ethical research involving humans.
- Key Principles:

- **Risk vs. Benefit:** Research risks must be justified by potential benefits.
- **Vulnerable Populations:** Extra care is required for those unable to give informed consent.
- **Scientific Validity:** Research must be based on sound scientific knowledge.

3. Belmont Report (1979):

- Developed in response to unethical studies like the Tuskegee Syphilis Study, where African American men were left untreated for syphilis to observe disease progression.
- Key Ethical Principles:
  - **Respect for Persons:** Protecting autonomy and providing special care for vulnerable individuals.
  - **Beneficence:** Maximizing benefits and minimizing risks.
  - **Justice:** Fair distribution of research benefits and burdens.

Principles Of Ethical Research

The Belmont Report's principles form the ethical foundation of clinical research:

1. Respect for Persons:

- Treat individuals as autonomous agents capable of making decisions about participation.
- Protect vulnerable populations such as children, pregnant women, prisoners, and individuals with cognitive impairments.

2. Beneficence:
- Obligation to minimize harm and maximize potential benefits.
- Requires a thorough risk-benefit analysis.

3. Justice:
- Fair distribution of research opportunities and burdens.
- Avoid exploitation of disadvantaged groups while ensuring access to research benefits for all.

Informed Consent

Informed consent is a process, not just a form, that ensures participants understand the study and voluntarily agree to take part.

Components of Informed Consent:

1. **Disclosure:**
   - Purpose, procedures, risks, benefits, and alternatives must be clearly explained.
   - Any potential conflicts of interest should be disclosed.

2. **Comprehension:**
   - Information must be presented in a language and format that the participant can understand.
   - Participants should be encouraged to ask questions.

3. **Voluntariness:**
   - Participation must be free from coercion or

undue influence.

Challenges in Informed Consent:

- **Language Barriers:** Ensuring comprehension among participants with different languages or literacy levels.
- **Cultural Sensitivity:** Respecting cultural norms without compromising ethical standards.
- **Complex Studies:** Simplifying technical information for participants to understand.

Role of Institutional Review Boards (IRBs)

IRBs, also known as Ethics Committees in some regions, are independent bodies responsible for ensuring research is conducted ethically.

1. Composition of IRBs:

- Multidisciplinary, including scientists, non-scientists, and community representatives.
- Must remain independent of the research being reviewed.

2. Functions of IRBs:

- **Review of Study Protocols:** Ensure studies are ethically sound and scientifically valid.
- **Risk-Benefit Assessment:** Evaluate whether participant risks are justified by potential benefits.
- **Informed Consent Review:** Confirm that consent processes are thorough and appropriate.
- **Monitoring Ongoing Research:** Conduct periodic reviews to ensure compliance with ethical standards.

3. Investigator Responsibilities to IRBs:

- Submit all required documents, including protocols

and informed consent forms.
- Report any adverse events, protocol deviations, or unanticipated problems.
- Provide updates for ongoing studies and apply for renewal approval if the study extends beyond initial timelines.

CHAPTER 3: STUDY DESIGN BASICS

Designing a robust study is critical for generating reliable and valid results.

Understanding Study Designs

Study designs are categorized based on the research question and methodology. The choice of design significantly influences the validity and generalizability of the findings.

1. Descriptive Studies:
- **Purpose:** To describe the characteristics of a population, disease, or phenomenon without exploring cause-effect relationships.
- **Examples:** Case reports, case series, cross-sectional studies.
- **Use Cases:** Estimating disease prevalence or demographic patterns.
- **Advantages:** Easy to conduct, provides valuable insights for hypothesis generation.
- **Limitations:** Cannot establish causation.

2. Analytical Studies:
- **Purpose:** To investigate associations between variables and potential causal relationships.
- **Types:**
  - **Cohort Studies:** Follow a group with

shared characteristics over time to observe outcomes.
- **Case-Control Studies:** Compare participants with a condition (cases) to those without (controls) to identify risk factors.
- **Advantages:** Useful for studying rare diseases or outcomes.
- **Limitations:** Susceptible to recall bias (case-control) or loss to follow-up (cohort).

3. Experimental Studies:
- **Purpose:** To test interventions under controlled conditions.
- **Examples:** Randomized Controlled Trials (RCTs).
- **Key Features:**
  - Randomization of participants.
  - Controlled settings to minimize confounding factors.
  - Blinding to reduce bias.
- **Advantages:** High internal validity, can establish causation.
- **Limitations:** Expensive, may lack external validity.

4. Quasi-Experimental Studies:
- **Purpose:** To evaluate interventions where randomization is not feasible.
- **Examples:** Before-and-after studies, interrupted time series.
- **Advantages:** Useful in real-world settings.
- **Limitations:** Greater risk of bias compared to RCTs.

Key Elements Of A Study Protocol

A study protocol is the blueprint for a research study. It ensures standardization, ethical compliance, and scientific rigor.

1. Objectives:
- Clearly defined primary and secondary objectives guide the study's focus.
- Example: Primary objective—assess the efficacy of a new antihypertensive drug in reducing blood pressure.

2. Hypothesis:
- A testable statement predicting the relationship between variables.
- Example: "The new antihypertensive drug reduces systolic blood pressure more effectively than placebo."

3. Methodology:
- Detailed description of the study design, sample size, intervention, and data collection methods.
- Example: A double-blind, placebo-controlled RCT with a parallel-group design.

4. Inclusion and Exclusion Criteria:
- **Inclusion Criteria:** Define who can participate (e.g., age range, diagnosis).
- **Exclusion Criteria:** Identify factors that disqualify participation (e.g., comorbid conditions).

5. Endpoints:
- Outcomes measured to evaluate the intervention's effect.
    - **Primary Endpoint:** The main outcome (e.g., reduction in blood pressure).
    - **Secondary Endpoint:** Additional outcomes of interest (e.g., quality of life).

Randomization And Blinding

1. Randomization:
Randomization ensures that participants are assigned to study groups without bias.

- **Purpose:**
    - Balances known and unknown confounding variables across groups.
    - Enhances the validity of causal inferences.
- **Techniques:**
    - **Simple Randomization:** Each participant has an equal chance of being assigned to any group.
    - **Stratified Randomization:** Ensures balance within subgroups (e.g., age, gender).
    - **Block Randomization:** Maintains equal group sizes within blocks.

2. Blinding:

Blinding reduces bias by concealing group assignments.

- **Types:**
    - **Single-Blind:** Only participants are unaware of group assignments.
    - **Double-Blind:** Both participants and researchers are unaware.
    - **Triple-Blind:** Participants, researchers, and data analysts are blinded.
- **Advantages:**
    - Prevents placebo effects and observer bias.
    - Ensures objective assessment of outcomes.

Bias In Research

Bias refers to systematic errors that distort study results. Recognizing and minimizing bias is crucial for ensuring the validity of findings.

1. Types of Bias:
- **Selection Bias:** Occurs when the study population is not representative of the target population.
  - Example: Recruiting only hospital patients for a study on a community disease.
- **Measurement Bias:** Results from inaccuracies in data collection.
  - Example: Using a faulty device to measure blood pressure.
- **Recall Bias:** Common in retrospective studies, where participants may misremember past events.
  - Example: Patients with lung cancer may overestimate past smoking habits.
- **Observer Bias:** When researchers' expectations influence data collection or interpretation.

2. Strategies to Minimize Bias:
- Use random sampling and randomization to prevent selection bias.
- Standardize measurement tools and procedures to avoid measurement bias.
- Train data collectors and employ objective data sources to reduce observer bias.
- Use blinding techniques to limit placebo effects and observer influences.

CHAPTER 4: DATA COLLECTION AND MANAGEMENT

Effective data collection and management are pivotal in clinical research, as they ensure the validity and reliability of the study's outcomes.

Data Collection Methods

Data collection methods vary depending on the study design and objectives.

Employing the right method is crucial for gathering relevant, accurate, and reliable data.

1. Surveys and Questionnaires:
- **Purpose:** Collect self-reported data from participants.
- **Advantages:**
    - Cost-effective and scalable for large populations.
    - Can be administered in various formats (paper, online, phone).
- **Limitations:**
    - Responses may be influenced by social desirability bias.
    - Poorly designed questions can yield unreliable data.

2. Interviews:
- **Purpose:** Gather in-depth qualitative data through direct interaction.

- **Types:**
  - Structured: Predefined questions with limited flexibility.
  - Semi-structured: Combines predefined questions with open-ended ones.
  - Unstructured: Exploratory with no predefined questions.
- **Advantages:**
  - Provides rich, detailed insights.
  - Allows clarification of ambiguous responses.
- **Limitations:**
  - Time-consuming and resource-intensive.
  - May introduce interviewer bias.

3. Medical Records:

- **Purpose:** Utilize existing clinical data for research purposes.
- **Advantages:**
  - Provides real-world, historical data.
  - Avoids burdening participants with additional procedures.
- **Limitations:**
  - Data quality depends on the accuracy of the original records.
  - Access may be restricted due to privacy concerns.

4. Laboratory Tests and Measurements:

- **Purpose:** Collect objective, measurable data on biological or physiological parameters.
- **Examples:** Blood tests, imaging studies, genetic testing.
- **Advantages:**

- Highly reliable and specific.
- Enables tracking of biomarkers and disease progression.
- **Limitations:**
  - Can be expensive and invasive.
  - Requires standardized protocols for consistency.

Developing Case Report Forms (Crfs)

Case Report Forms (CRFs) are tools used to capture study-specific data from participants. Proper CRF design is critical to ensuring data quality and consistency.

1. Essential Elements of CRFs:
- **Participant Information:** Unique identifiers, demographic details, and study-specific IDs.
- **Study Variables:** Clearly defined variables corresponding to the research objectives.
- **Data Collection Sections:** Organized to reflect the study's timeline (e.g., baseline, follow-up, endpoint).
- **Instructions for Data Collectors:** Ensure clarity on how to complete each section.

2. Common Mistakes in CRF Design:
- **Over-Complexity:** Including unnecessary fields that burden data collectors and analysts.
- **Ambiguous Questions:** Leading to inconsistent or incomplete responses.
- **Lack of Standardization:** Using varying formats or terminologies across forms.
- **Insufficient Piloting:** Failing to test CRFs can result in unanticipated issues during data collection.

Best Practices:

- Pilot CRFs on a small group of participants to identify potential problems.
- Use standardized terminologies (e.g., SNOMED, LOINC) to enhance clarity and interoperability.
- Involve all stakeholders, including investigators and data managers, in the design process.

Data Storage And Security

Maintaining the confidentiality, integrity, and availability of research data is vital for ethical and regulatory compliance.

1. Data Confidentiality:
- **De-identification:** Remove personal identifiers like names and addresses to protect participant anonymity.
- **Data Access Controls:** Restrict access to authorized personnel only.
- **Regulatory Compliance:**
  - **HIPAA (Health Insurance Portability and Accountability Act):** Governs the use and disclosure of protected health information in the U.S.
  - **GDPR (General Data Protection Regulation):** Provides comprehensive data protection rules for the European Union.

2. Data Storage:
- **Physical Storage:** Use locked cabinets for paper records in secure locations.
- **Electronic Storage:**

- Use encrypted databases with secure access protocols.
- Regularly back up data to prevent loss.
- Employ redundant systems to ensure data availability during failures.

3. Data Sharing:
   - Use secure file transfer methods and data sharing agreements to ensure responsible data use.
   - Anonymize datasets before sharing for secondary research.

Quality Assurance And Monitoring

Quality assurance (QA) and monitoring are processes designed to ensure that collected data is accurate, reliable, and compliant with the study protocol.

1. Quality Assurance:
   - **Standard Operating Procedures (SOPs):** Establish SOPs for all aspects of data collection and management.
   - **Training:** Ensure all personnel involved in data collection are properly trained.
   - **Data Validation:** Implement checks to identify and correct inconsistencies or errors in real time.

2. Monitoring:
   - **Purpose:** Ensure the study adheres to the protocol and that data collection processes meet predefined standards.
   - **Types of Monitoring:**
     - **On-Site Monitoring:** In-person visits to verify source data and CRF entries.
     - **Remote Monitoring:** Reviewing electronic records and reports from a distance.

- **Key Monitoring Activities:**
    - Verify informed consent documentation.
    - Check adherence to inclusion/exclusion criteria.
    - Assess data completeness and accuracy.

3. Auditing:
- Conduct periodic audits by independent parties to assess overall compliance and identify systemic issues.

CHAPTER 5: STATISTICAL FOUNDATIONS FOR BEGINNERS

Statistics is the backbone of clinical research, providing tools to analyze data and draw meaningful conclusions.

Basic Statistical Concepts

Understanding the basics of statistics is crucial for interpreting research data effectively.

1. Types of Data:

Data can be classified based on the nature of the variables being measured.

- **Nominal Data:**
    - **Definition:** Categorical data with no inherent order.
    - **Examples:** Gender (male/female), blood type (A, B, AB, O).
    - **Analysis:** Frequency counts, mode, chi-square tests.
- **Ordinal Data:**
    - **Definition:** Categorical data with a meaningful order but no fixed intervals.
    - **Examples:** Pain scale (mild, moderate, severe), Likert scale responses.
    - **Analysis:** Median, non-parametric tests like Mann-Whitney U test.
- **Interval Data:**
    - **Definition:** Numeric data with equal

intervals between values but no true zero.
- **Examples:** Temperature in Celsius or Fahrenheit.
- **Analysis:** Mean, standard deviation, correlation.
- **Ratio Data:**
  - **Definition:** Numeric data with a true zero point, allowing for meaningful ratios.
  - **Examples:** Weight, height, blood pressure.
  - **Analysis:** Mean, t-tests, regression analysis.

2. Measures of Central Tendency:

These describe the center or typical value in a dataset.

- **Mean (Average):** Sum of all values divided by the total number of observations.
- **Median:** The middle value when data is ordered.
- **Mode:** The most frequently occurring value(s).

3. Measures of Variability:

These describe the spread or dispersion of data.

- **Range:** Difference between the highest and lowest values.
- **Variance:** The average squared deviation from the mean.
- **Standard Deviation (SD):** The square root of variance, indicating the average deviation from the mean.
- **Interquartile Range (IQR):** The range of the middle 50% of data (difference between the 25th and 75th percentiles).

Study Power And Sample Size

1. Importance of Study Power:

- **Definition:** The probability of detecting a true effect or difference when one exists.
- **Factors Influencing Power:**
    - Sample size: Larger samples increase power.
    - Effect size: Larger differences are easier to detect.
    - Significance level (alpha): Lower alpha reduces the chance of false positives but decreases power.

2. Sample Size Calculation Basics:
Determining an adequate sample size is critical for study validity.

- **Steps in Sample Size Calculation:**
    - Define the primary outcome measure.
    - Estimate the expected effect size.
    - Choose a significance level (e.g., 0.05) and desired power (e.g., 80% or 90%).
    - Use statistical formulas or software to calculate sample size.
- **Common Tools for Calculation:**
    - Online calculators.
    - Statistical software like G*Power or R.

Commonly Used Statistical Tests

Statistical tests help analyze relationships and differences in data. Choosing the right test depends on the data type and study design.

1. T-Tests:
- **Purpose:** Compare means between two groups.
- **Types:**
    - **Independent t-test:** For two unrelated groups (e.g., treatment vs. control).

- **Paired t-test:** For related groups (e.g., pre-treatment vs. post-treatment in the same participants).

2. Chi-Square Test:
- **Purpose:** Assess associations between categorical variables.
- **Example:** Comparing proportions of males and females with a specific disease.

3. Analysis of Variance (ANOVA):
- **Purpose:** Compare means across three or more groups.
- **Types:**
    - **One-way ANOVA:** One independent variable (e.g., drug doses).
    - **Two-way ANOVA:** Two independent variables (e.g., drug doses and age groups).

4. Correlation:
- **Purpose:** Measure the strength and direction of a relationship between two continuous variables.
- **Common Correlation Coefficients:**
    - **Pearson's r:** For normally distributed data.
    - **Spearman's rho:** For non-parametric data.

Introduction To Statistical Software

Statistical software simplifies data analysis and helps researchers perform complex calculations efficiently.

1. SPSS (Statistical Package for the Social Sciences):
- **Overview:** Widely used for social sciences and healthcare research.
- **Strengths:**

- User-friendly interface with point-and-click functionality.
- Comprehensive range of statistical tests.
  - **Limitations:**
    - Requires a license, which can be expensive.

2. **R:**
   - **Overview:** A free, open-source software environment for statistical computing and graphics.
   - **Strengths:**
     - Highly customizable through packages.
     - Excellent for advanced analyses and visualizations.
   - **Limitations:**
     - Steeper learning curve for beginners.

3. **Excel:**
   - **Overview:** Commonly used spreadsheet software with basic statistical functions.
   - **Strengths:**
     - Easily accessible and familiar to most users.
     - Suitable for small datasets and simple analyses.
   - **Limitations:**
     - Limited advanced statistical capabilities.
     - Prone to errors in complex analyses without add-ins.

Getting Started With Statistical Software:

- **SPSS:** Start with descriptive statistics, t-tests, and chi-

square tests.
- **R:** Learn basic commands like summary(), plot(), and use RStudio for a user-friendly interface.
- **Excel:** Use formulas like =AVERAGE(), =STDEV(), and =CORREL() for initial exploration.

CHAPTER 6: WRITING AND PUBLISHING YOUR RESEARCH

Writing and publishing a research paper is a critical step in sharing findings with the scientific community and advancing medical knowledge.

How To Write A Research Paper

A well-structured research paper conveys the study's objectives, methodology, findings, and implications.

The IMRaD format—**Introduction, Methods, Results, and Discussion**—is widely used in scientific writing.

1. **IMRaD Structure:**
   - **Introduction:**
     - **Purpose:** Explain the research question and its significance.
     - **Key Elements:**
       - Background and context: What is already known?
       - Knowledge gap: What is missing in current research?
       - Objective: What does the study aim to achieve?

     Example: "Despite advances in therapy, the optimal management of [condition] remains unclear. This study aims to evaluate [specific intervention] in improving [outcomes]."

- **Methods:**
  - **Purpose:** Provide a clear, reproducible description of how the study was conducted.
  - **Key Elements:**
    - Study design: Specify the type (e.g., RCT, cohort study).
    - Population: Describe inclusion/exclusion criteria.
    - Procedures: Detail interventions, measurements, and data collection methods.
    - Statistical analysis: Mention software and tests used.

Example: "Participants were randomly assigned to receive [intervention] or [control]. Primary outcomes were measured using [specific tool]. Data were analyzed using SPSS version 25."

- **Results:**
  - **Purpose:** Present findings objectively.
  - **Key Elements:**
    - Use tables and figures to summarize data.
    - Report primary and secondary outcomes.
    - Avoid interpretation—save that for the Discussion.

Example: "The intervention group showed a significant improvement in [outcome] compared to the control group ($p = 0.03$)."

- **Discussion:**
  - **Purpose:** Interpret the findings in context.
  - **Key Elements:**

- Compare results to previous studies.
- Discuss strengths, limitations, and implications.
- Suggest future research directions.

Example: "Our findings support the use of [intervention] in [condition]. However, the study was limited by [limitation], suggesting the need for larger trials."

Choosing The Right Journal

Selecting an appropriate journal increases the likelihood of publication and ensures your research reaches the intended audience.

1. Factors to Consider:
- **Journal Scope:** Ensure the topic aligns with the journal's focus.
- **Target Audience:** Identify whether the journal caters to clinicians, researchers, or a specific specialty.
- **Impact Factor:** Consider journals with a high impact factor for significant findings.
- **Open Access vs. Subscription-Based Journals:** Open-access journals have wider reach but may charge publication fees.

2. How to Identify Potential Journals:
- Use tools like Elsevier's *Journal Finder* or Springer's *Journal Suggester*.
- Review journals cited in your references for relevance.
- Read the journal's "Instructions for Authors" for submission guidelines.

The Peer Review Process

Peer review ensures research quality and validity. Understanding the process helps authors navigate it effectively.

1. What to Expect:
- **Initial Screening:** The editor assesses the manuscript for relevance and quality.
- **Review by Experts:** Subject matter experts evaluate the study's methodology, analysis, and significance.
- **Feedback:** Reviewers provide comments and recommend acceptance, revision, or rejection.

2. Responding to Reviewer Comments:
- Be professional and objective, even when critiques seem harsh.
- Address each comment in detail, referencing changes made in the revised manuscript.
- If you disagree, provide a clear, evidence-based rationale.

Example Response: "We appreciate the reviewer's suggestion regarding [aspect]. We have revised [section] accordingly (see page X). Alternatively, we believe that [specific rationale] supports our original approach."

Ethical Issues In Publication

Ethical considerations ensure the integrity of scientific literature and protect researchers' and participants' rights.

1. Avoiding Plagiarism:
- **Definition:** Using others' ideas or words without proper attribution.
- **Prevention:**
  - Cite all sources accurately.
  - Use plagiarism detection software like

Turnitin or iThenticate.

2. **Ensuring Authorship Integrity:**
   - **Criteria for Authorship (ICMJE Guidelines):**
     - Substantial contributions to study conception, design, data analysis, or interpretation.
     - Drafting or revising the manuscript critically.
     - Final approval of the version to be published.
     - Accountability for all aspects of the work.

3. **Other Ethical Considerations:**
   - **Duplicate Submission:** Avoid submitting the same manuscript to multiple journals.
   - **Data Fabrication and Falsification:** Present only accurate and verified data.
   - **Conflict of Interest:** Disclose financial or personal relationships that could bias the study.

Example Disclosure: "The authors declare no conflicts of interest related to this study."

CHAPTER 7: CHALLENGES AND PITFALLS IN CLINICAL RESEARCH

Clinical research, while rewarding, presents numerous challenges, particularly for beginners. Addressing these obstacles effectively is critical for the success and integrity of a study.

Common Challenges For Beginners

Starting a clinical research project can be daunting due to resource constraints, logistical difficulties, and knowledge gaps.

1. **Funding**
   - **Challenges:**
     - Limited access to grants or institutional support.
     - Competition for funding from government agencies or private sponsors.
   - **Solutions:**
     - Start with small pilot studies that require fewer resources.
     - Explore alternative funding sources, such as crowdfunding, industry partnerships, or institutional seed grants.
     - Develop a detailed and realistic budget proposal to increase your chances of securing funding.

Example: A novice researcher successfully obtained funding by applying to a local health organization for a project targeting community health needs.

2. Recruitment

- **Challenges:**
    - Identifying eligible participants.
    - Convincing individuals to enroll while addressing concerns about risks or time commitments.
    - Maintaining participant retention.
- **Solutions:**
    - Use multiple recruitment strategies: advertisements, community outreach, and collaboration with healthcare providers.
    - Simplify the study process for participants, offering flexible scheduling and clear communication.
    - Provide incentives like transportation reimbursements or small monetary compensation.

Example: A study faced recruitment delays but overcame them by partnering with local clinics to reach more potential participants.

3. Time Management

- **Challenges:**
    - Balancing research with clinical, teaching, or administrative responsibilities.
    - Delays in approvals, data collection, or analysis.
- **Solutions:**

- Develop a clear timeline with milestones.
- Delegate tasks to research assistants or team members.
- Use project management tools like Trello or Gantt charts to track progress.

Avoiding Misconduct

Ethical breaches, whether intentional or accidental, can jeopardize a study's credibility and lead to severe consequences.

1. Types of Misconduct:
- **Fabrication:** Inventing data or results.
- **Falsification:** Manipulating research materials, processes, or data.
- **Plagiarism:** Using another's work or ideas without proper attribution.

2. Strategies to Prevent Misconduct:
- **Training:** Ensure all team members understand ethical guidelines like those outlined in Good Clinical Practice (GCP).
- **Data Management:** Implement systems to secure raw data, such as electronic data capture (EDC) platforms with audit trails.
- **Accountability:** Foster a culture of transparency by regularly reviewing data and progress.

Case Study:
- **Scenario:** A researcher manipulated data to align with expected outcomes, which was later discovered during

peer review.
- **Lesson Learned:** Strict data validation protocols and periodic audits could have prevented this issue.

3. **Reporting Misconduct:**
   - Encourage whistleblowing mechanisms where team members can report concerns confidentially.
   - Follow institutional policies for investigating allegations of misconduct.

Learning From Failures

Failures and mistakes are inevitable but provide valuable lessons for improving future research practices.

1. Case Study: Recruitment Failure

- **Scenario:** A researcher's study aimed to recruit 200 participants for a clinical trial but enrolled only 50 due to overly restrictive inclusion criteria and poor outreach.
- **Solution:** The team revised criteria to widen eligibility and engaged with community leaders to enhance recruitment efforts.
- **Takeaway:** Plan recruitment strategies early, and regularly assess progress against goals.

2. Case Study: Data Loss

- **Scenario:** A small clinical trial lost months of data when a laptop containing raw files was stolen.
- **Solution:** The team switched to a secure cloud-based storage system and mandated regular backups.
- **Takeaway:** Use secure, redundant systems for data

storage and implement data management best practices.

3. Case Study: Protocol Deviation

- **Scenario:** A research assistant accidentally administered the wrong dosage of an intervention in a randomized trial, violating the study protocol.
- **Solution:** The team retrained all staff, revised workflows to include dose verification steps, and reported the deviation to the Institutional Review Board (IRB).
- **Takeaway:** Conduct regular training and audits to ensure adherence to protocols.

4. Case Study: Statistical Misinterpretation

- **Scenario:** A published study reported significant findings due to a miscalculated p-value, which was later corrected by an independent statistician.
- **Solution:** The research team consulted a biostatistician for future studies and validated all analyses before submission.
- **Takeaway:** Collaborate with experts to ensure accuracy in data analysis.

CHAPTER 8: FUTURE TRENDS IN CLINICAL RESEARCH

The landscape of clinical research is evolving rapidly, driven by technological advancements, innovative methodologies, and a growing emphasis on personalized care.

Emerging Technologies

Technological innovations are transforming how clinical trials are designed, conducted, and analyzed.

1. Artificial Intelligence (AI)
    - **Applications:**
        - **Data Analysis:** AI can process vast datasets quickly, identifying patterns and insights that might be missed using traditional methods.
        - **Patient Recruitment:** Algorithms analyze electronic health records (EHRs) to identify eligible participants efficiently.
        - **Predictive Modeling:** AI forecasts trial outcomes, optimizing resource allocation.
    - **Challenges:**
        - Regulatory frameworks for AI in clinical research are still developing.
        - Ethical concerns about algorithm transparency and bias.
    - **Example:** AI-driven tools like IBM Watson Health are

being used to design precision oncology trials.

2. Big Data

- **Definition:** The collection and analysis of large, complex datasets from diverse sources, including EHRs, wearables, social media, and genomic databases.
- **Impact on Research:**
  - Enables researchers to analyze real-world evidence and trends.
  - Supports longitudinal studies by providing continuous data streams.
- **Example:** The All of Us Research Program uses big data to study diverse populations and develop tailored treatments.

3. Real-World Evidence (Rwe)

- **Definition:** Data collected outside controlled trial settings, such as from routine clinical practice, patient registries, or wearable devices.
- **Impact:**
  - Complements traditional clinical trial data.
  - Helps assess drug effectiveness in diverse populations and long-term outcomes.
- **Challenges:**
  - Ensuring data quality and consistency across sources.

Decentralized Clinical Trials

Decentralized trials (DCTs) leverage technology to conduct research remotely, offering greater accessibility and convenience for participants.

1. **Telemedicine**
    - **Applications:**
        - Virtual consultations for participant screening and follow-up.
        - Remote monitoring of patient-reported outcomes.
    - **Benefits:**
        - Reduces the need for site visits, enhancing participation from diverse populations.
        - Saves time and resources for both participants and researchers.
    - **Challenges:**
        - Ensuring compliance with regulatory requirements for remote data collection.
        - Addressing digital access disparities among participants.

2. Virtual Research Platforms

- **Definition:** Online systems that manage all aspects of a trial, from recruitment to data analysis.
- **Features:**
    - Real-time data sharing and monitoring.
    - Integration with electronic health records and wearable devices.
- **Example:** Platforms like Medable and Science 37 facilitate fully virtual clinical trials.

3. Wearables And Mobile Health (Mhealth) Devices

- **Applications:**
  - Continuous monitoring of vital signs, activity levels, and medication adherence.
  - Collecting real-time data to assess intervention effects.
- **Benefits:**
  - Provides richer datasets with fewer disruptions to participants' daily lives.
  - Enhances study adherence and engagement.
- **Challenges:**
  - Standardizing data formats and ensuring device accuracy.

Personalized Medicine

Personalized medicine tailors healthcare interventions to individual genetic, environmental, and lifestyle factors, significantly impacting clinical research.

1. Impact on Trial Design

- **Stratified Trials:** Subgroup analyses based on genetic or molecular markers.
- **Adaptive Designs:** Trials that evolve based on interim data, allowing for modifications to treatment arms or patient eligibility.
- **N-of-1 Trials:** Single-patient studies evaluating individualized treatment responses.
- **Example:** Basket trials and umbrella trials in oncology, where treatments are matched to molecular profiles rather than tumor location.

2. Genomics and Biomarker Research
- **Role:** Identifying biomarkers enables the development of targeted therapies and precision diagnostics.
- **Example:** The use of HER2 biomarkers in breast cancer to guide trastuzumab treatment.

3. Challenges:
- High costs of genomic and molecular testing.
- Ethical concerns about genetic privacy and discrimination.

APPENDICES

Glossary Of Clinical Research Terms

- **Adverse Event (AE):** Any undesirable experience associated with the use of a medical product in a patient.
- **Blinding:** A method to prevent bias in a trial by keeping participants, investigators, or both unaware of the assigned treatment groups.
- **Clinical Trial:** A research study designed to evaluate the safety and efficacy of medical, surgical, or behavioral interventions.
- **Cohort Study:** An observational study where participants with shared characteristics are followed over time to observe outcomes.
- **Data Monitoring Committee (DMC):** An independent group that monitors data during a clinical trial to ensure participant safety.
- **Informed Consent:** A process by which participants voluntarily confirm their willingness to participate in a study after being informed of all aspects of the trial.
- **Randomization:** Assigning participants to different groups in a trial using a random process to reduce bias.
- **Standard Operating Procedures (SOPs):** Detailed, written instructions to achieve uniformity in the performance of specific functions.

Templates And Checklists

1. Study Protocol Template

A standardized structure for documenting all aspects of a clinical study.

Sample Outline:
- **Title Page:** Study title, identifiers, version, and date.
- **Background and Rationale:** Scientific basis and justification.
- **Objectives and Hypotheses:** Clearly defined aims and expected outcomes.
- **Methodology:** Study design, sample size, interventions, and data collection methods.
- **Inclusion/Exclusion Criteria:** Eligibility requirements for participants.
- **Ethical Considerations:** IRB approval, informed consent process.
- **Statistical Analysis Plan:** Methods for analyzing collected data.

2. Informed Consent Form Template

A comprehensive form ensuring participants understand the study's purpose, risks, and benefits.

Key Sections:
- Study purpose and description.
- Potential risks and benefits.
- Confidentiality and data usage.
- Voluntary participation and withdrawal rights.

3. Data Management Checklist

To ensure data integrity, security, and compliance with regulatory standards:

- Verify all data collection tools (e.g., CRFs, electronic systems).
- Implement secure data storage solutions.
- Define data validation procedures.
- Conduct regular audits for accuracy and completeness.

Additional Resources

Expand your knowledge and skills with these curated resources:
Books:

- *Designing Clinical Research* by Stephen B. Hulley et al.
- *Fundamentals of Clinical Trials* by Lawrence M. Friedman et al.
- *Practical Statistics for Medical Research* by Douglas G. Altman.

Websites:

- ClinicalTrials.gov: Database of publicly and privately funded clinical studies.
- ICH GCP Guidelines: International standards for Good Clinical Practice.
- NIH Office of Extramural Research: Resources on clinical trial funding and management.

Online Courses:

- **Introduction to Clinical Research:** Available on Coursera or edX.
- **Good Clinical Practice (GCP) Training:** Offered by TransCelerate BioPharma and NIH.
- **Biostatistics in Clinical Research:** Found on platforms like FutureLearn or Udemy.

ABOUT THE AUTHOR

Dr Essam Abdelhakim

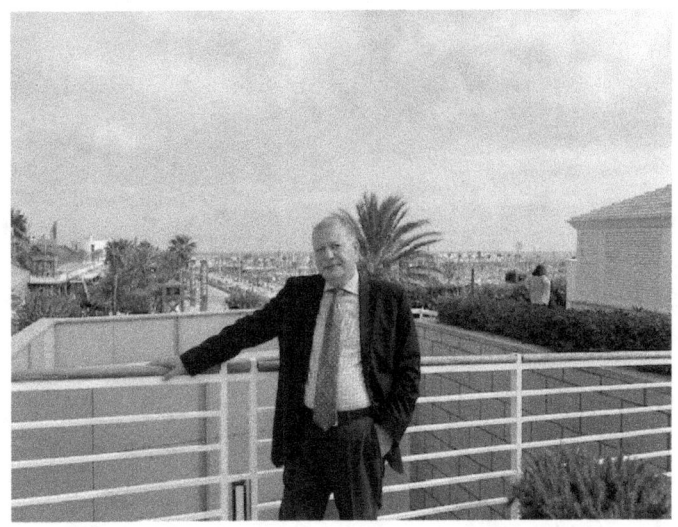

Senior Investigator and Expert in Clinical research

www.ingramcontent.com/pod-product-compliance
Lightning Source LLC
Chambersburg PA
CBHW070941220526
45469CB00007B/2469